How to thrive intermittent fasting for women

A woman comprehensive handbook guide

By

Donovan Alston

Table of content

Introduction

Irregular fasting has turned into an undeniably famous wellbeing pattern, as it offers a novel way to deal with weight reduction and, generally, prosperity. By following a particular eating design that shifts back and forth among fasting and eating windows, people might possibly receive various rewards for both their physical and emotional well-being. In this thorough guide, we will dive into the universe of irregular fasting, investigating different techniques, procedures, and tips on the best way to successfully flourish with this way of life. Whether you are a novice hoping to kick off your excursion or somebody trying to improve their discontinuous fasting experience, this guide will give you important bits of knowledge and viable exhortation that will engage you to integrate irregular fasting into your everyday schedule effectively. Prepare to set out on a groundbreaking excursion towards better

Chapter 1

Prologue to discontinuous fasting for ladies

Discontinuous fasting is an eating plan that switches between fasting and eating on a normal schedule. Research shows that discontinuous fasting is a method for dealing with your weight and preventing — or even reversing — a few types of infection. Yet, how would you make it happen? Furthermore, is it safe?

What is irregular fasting?

Many weight-control plans center around what to eat, yet irregular fasting is about when you eat.

With irregular fasting, you just eat at a particular time. Research shows fasting for a specific number of hours every day or eating only one, two, or three days a week might have medical advantages.

Johns Hopkins neuroscientist Imprint Mattson has studied discontinuous fasting for a considerable length of time. He says our bodies have advanced enough to have the option to go without nourishment for a long time, or even a few days or longer. In ancient times, before people figured out how to cultivate, they were trackers and finders who developed the ability to get by—and flourish—for extensive stretches without eating. The process of chasing game and assembling nuts and berries required significant investment. In the US, maintaining sound load was simpler, with no network programs and people not eating after a workout. Segments were smaller, and more people worked and played outside, leading to increased activity.

With the web, television, and other diversion accessible every minute of every day, numerous adults and youngsters stay alert for longer hours to stare at the television, look at virtual entertainment, mess around, and visit the web. That can mean sitting and nibbling the entire day—and the greater part of the evening.

Additional calories and less action can mean a higher risk of stoutness, type 2 diabetes, coronary illness, and other diseases. Logical examinations are showing that irregular fasting might assist with switching these patterns.

How does irregular fasting function?

Regular fasting is a method of eating and fasting that involves choosing specific time periods to eat and fast. Some examples include eating only during an eight-hour period daily and fasting for the rest of the week, or eating a single dinner daily, two days a week. Mattson explains that without food at night, the body depletes its sugar stores and starts consuming fat, referred to as metabolic exchange. This differs from the typical American eating pattern, where people consume all their meals and snacks without exercising. Discontinuous fasting works by reducing the time when the body has consumed the calories from the last meal and starts consuming fat.

Irregular Fasting Plans

It means quite a bit to check with your primary care physician prior to beginning irregular fasting. When you receive their approval, the genuine practice is straightforward. You can pick an everyday methodology, which confines day-to-day eating to one six- to eight-hour time frame every day. Albeit certain individuals find it simple to stay with this example over the long haul, one exploration that was not planned explicitly to take a gander at an irregular fasting design found that restricting your everyday time window of eating doesn't forestall weight gain over the long run or yield huge weight reduction results. That study's outcomes showed that decreasing the quantity of huge feasts or eating all the smaller dinners might be related to limiting weight gain or even weight reduction over the long run.

One more discontinuous fasting plan, known as the 5:2 methodology, includes eating consistently five days a week. For the other two days, you restrict yourself to one 500–600 calorie feast. A model would be in the event that you decided to eat typically on each day of the week with the exception of Mondays and Thursdays, which would be your one-feast days.

Longer periods without food, like 24-, 36-, 48-, and 72-hour fasting periods, are not really better for you and might be perilous. Going excessively long without eating could really urge your body to begin putting away more fat because of starvation.

Mattson's examination demonstrates the way that it can take two to about a month before the body becomes familiar with discontinuous fasting. You could feel eager or grouchy while you're becoming accustomed to the new everyday practice. However, he notices that research subjects who endure the change in time frame will generally stay with the arrangement since they notice they feel improved.

What could I eat at any point while discontinuous fasting?

During your eating periods, "eating ordinarily" doesn't mean going off the deep end. Research shows that you're not prone to getting more fit or getting better assuming you pack your meals with unhealthy, low-quality food, super-sized broiled things, and treats.

Yet, a few specialists like irregular fasting because it takes into consideration a range of various food sources to be eaten—and delighted in. Sharing great, nutritious food with others and relishing the suppertime experience adds fulfillment and supports great wellbeing.

Most nutrition specialists view the Mediterranean eating routine as a decent outline of what to eat, regardless of whether you're attempting discontinuous fasting. You can barely turn out badly when you pick salad greens, solid fats, lean protein, and mind-boggling raw carbs like entire grains.

Irregular Fasting Advantages

Research shows that irregular fasting periods accomplish more than consuming fat. One of "Numerous things occur during discontinuous fasting that can safeguard organs against persistent sicknesses like type 2 diabetes, coronary illness, age-related neurodegenerative issues, even provocative entrail infections, and numerous tumors," he says.

Here are some discontinuous fasting benefits that research has uncovered up to this point:

Investigating the advantages intended for ladies wellbeing and health

Understanding Ladies' Wellbeing and Hormonal Equilibrium In this part, we'll give an outline of ladies' wellbeing and the meaning of hormonal equilibrium for general prosperity. Understanding the interesting difficulties and worries that ladies face will lay the groundwork for investigating how cardamom can be helpful.

Hormonal Equilibrium: Investigate the role of chemicals, like estrogen and progesterone, in ladies' wellbeing and essentialness. Comprehend the significance of keeping up with hormonal equilibrium for feminine wellbeing, regenerative capability, temperament solidity, and, by and large, health.

Everyday people's wellbeing concerns: Examine common wellbeing worries among ladies, like feminine inconsistencies, hormonal uneven characters, premenstrual disorder, menopausal side effects, and regenerative wellbeing. Perceive the possible effect of cardamom on tending to these worries.

Cardamom's Likely Advantages for Ladies' Hormonal Wellbeing

In this part, we'll dig into cardamom's possible advantages for ladies' hormonal wellbeing and prosperity. From conventional information to logical exploration, we'll reveal the possible components by which cardamom might uphold ladies' hormonal equilibrium.

Adjusting Chemicals: Find out how cardamom's regular mixtures, including phytoestrogens, may assist with supporting chemical guidelines and equilibrium. Investigate the likely impacts of cardamom on feminine consistency, mitigating feminine issues, decreasing PMS side effects, and advancing regenerative wellbeing.

Menopausal Help: Examine the capability of cardamom to alleviate menopausal side effects, for example, hot flashes, night sweats, temperament swings, and rest unsettling influences. Investigate cardamom's capability to help ladies during this temporary period of life and advance hormonal balance.

Cardamom for Stomach-Related Wellbeing and Prosperity

We'll investigate cardamom's expected advantages for ladies' stomach-related wellbeing, as legitimate processing assumes a vital part in overall prosperity.

Mitigating the Stomach-Related Framework: Find out how cardamom's medicinal balms, for example, cineole and terpinen-4-old, can assist with calming the stomach-related framework and ease normal stomach-related protests like swelling, heartburn, gas, and stomach inconvenience. Cardamom's carminative properties can advance solid absorption and reduce gastrointestinal trouble.

Supporting Solid Stomach Verdure: Investigate cardamom's capability to promote a good arrangement of stomach microorganisms. The antimicrobial properties of cardamom might assist with keeping an agreeable stomach microbiome, forestall harmful microscopic

organisms in excess, and advance
stomach-related health

wellbeing and essentialness with irregular
fasting!

Chapter 2:

wellbeing and essentialness with irregular fasting!

Irregular fasting (IF) includes cycling between times of eating and fasting. There are a few ways to deal with IF, each with its own fasting and eating windows. Here are some normal ones: 16/8 Technique: This includes fasting for 16 hours per day and eating within an 8-hour window. For instance, you could skip breakfast and eat from 12:00 PM to 8:00 PM. 5:2 Diet: In this methodology, you typically eat for five days every week and confine calorie intake to around 500–600 calories on the other two non-successful days. Eat-Stop-Eat: This strategy includes fasting for an entire 24 hours a few times per week. For example, you could fast from supper one day until supper the following day. Alternate-Day Fasting: As the name suggests, you shift back and forth between long periods of standard eating and long periods of extremely low-calorie consumption, or fasting. Warrior Diet: This approach includes eating limited quantities of crude products of the soil during the day and having one huge feast in the evening. OMAD (One Feast a Day): With OMAD, you fast for 23 hours and consume all your everyday calories in a single enormous dinner, as a rule, at dinner. The 5:25 Convention: This is a fresher methodology that joins a short 5-hour eating window with a 25-hour quick, giving adaptability in feast timing. Crescendo Technique: This strategy includes discontinuous fasting on non-successful days. For instance, fasting on Mondays, Wednesdays, and Fridays while eating regularly on other days Time-Constrained Eating (TRE): TRE is a more adaptable methodology where you pick an everyday fasting window that suits your schedule, like fasting for 14–18 hours. Extended Fasting: This includes fasting for longer periods, going from 48 hours to a few days. It ought to be finished under clinical supervision. Remember that the viability of these methodologies can vary from one individual to another. It's fundamental to talk with a medical professional prior to beginning any fasting routine, particularly on the off chance that you have a basic medical issue. Furthermore, remain hydrated and center around adjusted nourishment while practicing irregular fasting.

outline of well-known discontinuous fasting conventions

Discontinuous fasting

Discontinuous fasting is, in fact, not an eating plan but an approach to eating that focuses on the timing as opposed to the sort of food sources. Destining implies consuming very few to no calories for a while. There are various ways to deal with discontinuous fasting, and most normal regimens incorporate time-confined taking care of (restricting the "eating window" to 6–8 hours consistently), substitute day fasting (one day of fasting and one day of off-the-cuff taking care of), and occasional fasting (fasting for 1-2 days every week). With the growing interest in irregular fasting in general society,

more analysts have been analyzing the impacts
of discontinuous fasting on type 2 diabetes.
Current evidence shows reliable proof that
irregular fasting can assist with weight reduction
(through caloric limitation), yet there have been
mixed outcomes for upgrades in HbA1c, insulin
responsiveness, and other glycemic control
markers. While more exploration is required on
this subject, discontinuous fasting can be
prescribed to individuals who wish to achieve
their desired body weight, as weight reduction is
additionally regularly suggested for type 2
diabetes. While discontinuous fasting doesn't
give rules on the kinds of food varieties to
devour, individuals can integrate a smart dieting
design, as examined above, into their irregular
fasting routine to guarantee the nature of their
eating regimens. Once more, individuals who
intend to follow this eating technique ought to
work intimately with an expert to coordinate
insulin and medicine dosing with their eating
and fasting periods to accomplish ideal glycemic
control. In spite of the fact that water and
non-caloric fluids are permitted during fasting

periods, many individuals will generally drink less liquid on their fasting days. In this manner, to forestall dryness and hypotension, patients ought to be encouraged to drink sufficient fluids, decrease their diuretics, and be hostile to hypertensive medications during fasting periods.

Calorie Limitation in People

Discontinuous Fasting

Discontinuous fasting or times of forbearance from food and drink have been a typical strict practice since ancient times. Discontinuous fasting for the purpose of caloric limitation is gaining in prevalence. In research, discontinuous fasting has enveloped different regimens, including substitute day fasting (AFD), altered AFD, and the 5:2 eating routine [6]. AFD, which has accomplished a lot of logical concentration, comprises a day of not obligatory eating frequently alluded to as the "feed day," followed by a day with no caloric utilization called the "quick day. This rotating example of food admission goes on however long the dietary intercession would last. Changes to this severe system of taking care of and fasting were created with the mentality of working with a more elevated level of individual adherence over longer terms. Adjusted AFD, regularly alluded to in the writing as substitute day changed quick or ADMF, considers some caloric admission on the quick day, however seriously confined (75% caloric limitation). The 5:2 eating routine, or the Quick Eating Regime, endorses just 2 days of serious caloric limitation each week. Through these differing techniques for irregular fasting, the degree of caloric limitation accomplished can be compared to conventional caloric limitation programs; however, simplicity of execution (less calorie counting) and further developed long-haul consistency are apparent with discontinuous fasting. Gorging on the "feed day" because of raised hunger followed on from the "quick day" is clearly a worry with these methodologies. In any case, those who concentrate on discontinuous fasting have reasoned that even subsequent to fasting each and every other day, members report no compensatory eating and elevated degrees of satiety all through the length of the review. This perception likely mirrors a transformation to the discontinuous fasting routine accomplished within half a month [7]. Generally speaking, irregular fasting is novel and a possibly stronger mediation for weight reduction, protection of lean mass, and metabolic wellbeing in people. As far as anyone is concerned, there is just a single report that was intended to test the impacts of substitute day benefiting from nourishment in matures. Named the Appetite Study, 60 men, after exchanging long stretches of fasting and taking care of themselves, got a normal of 1500 kcal each day for quite some time, which added up to roughly 35% CR. The 60 different men were taken care of, but it was not obligatory. The underlying report from this study was brief, but examinations directed quite a while later [8] demonstrated that the demise rate would in general be brought down in the discontinuous fasting gathering, and emergency clinic confirmations decreased in these people by roughly half (123 days for CR versus 219 days for control). Concentrates on the contrast between irregular fasting and conventional CR for the capacity of discontinuous fasting to lessen age-related illness.

get sound, and truth be told, many eating regimens that cut out whole nutrition classes are undesirable. Your body needs a good arrangement of supplements, including sound fats and carbs. Finding a wholesome equilibrium that works for you will assist you in remaining persuaded and incorporating reasonable change into your life.

Picking the right strategy for your way of life and objectives

Making maintainable lifestyle changes is an interaction that requires some investment, commitment, and tolerance. Clinicians have found that it takes a normal of 66 days for another propensity to become programmed; however, actually constructing and keeping up with way of life changes is exceptionally difficult for every person. Thus, it is essential to set up your way of life to work with your life and to give yourself beauty as you track down the beat that works for you. Nonetheless, there are a few simple techniques that can assist you in fostering a lifestyle change plan that works for you.

Center around the entire picture.

Way of life changes resemble a riddle. There are many pieces that should make up the entire picture. Building propensities in only one region of the riddle will leave your general picture lacking. Your physical, mental, and profound wellbeing all work together to make and break way of life changes, so it is essential to comprehend how they all interface while setting up your way of life change plan.

Rest: The typical grownup ought to attempt to rest for 7-9 hours every evening. During a relaxing rest, you have the opportunity and energy to recover and re-energize. This time is vital to the outcome of making a way of life change. Absence of rest can bring about crabbiness, desires, and exhaustion, all of which can crash a fruitful way of life change.

Water: Hydration is the way to the majority of your important physical processes. Without remaining hydrated, neither your body nor your brain will be working with the lifestyle change process. In this way, get a major water container and hydrate!

Stress: By dealing with your body, you are normally indicating to your mind that your general feelings of anxiety can diminish. Another propensity can build up your pressure on the board framework and, at last, generally pressure the executive's achievement. Center around finding reasonable propensities you can incorporate into your daily schedule. You can expand on areas of strength for those schedules as you keep going after your drawn-out objectives.

 At the point when we fuel ourselves with unhealthy food, we will definitely crash and tumble off the way of life change cart. Center around tracking down solid trades for unhealthy food that you can really maintain.

Work out. Remaining dynamic influences your physical and emotional well-being. By tracking down fun ways of remaining dynamic, you give yourself extra endorphins that assist your cerebrum and body in working at maximum efficiency!

Put forth practical and feasible objectives.

The objectives you set for yourself are vital to your general outcome in changing your way of life. Center around putting forth objectives that are practical. Rather than hoping to run a long-distance race in a half-year, go for running a 5K and warm up for the long-distance race. Defining sensible objectives that you can accomplish and then expanding on them will assist you with keeping up with force and remaining roused.

Make everyday organized exercises connected with the

objectives

Incorporating exercises into your day helps you remain focused on your objectives. Rather than accepting that you will sort it out at the time, plan fun exercises you can anticipate over the course of the day that relate to your objective!

Make propensities that you can keep.

For the vast majority, it is unreasonable to accept that you will continuously be inspired. Thus, contemplate how you can construct propensities that are practical in your life, in any event, when you're not on the wellbeing kick. Figuring out how to trade out unhealthy food for better choices is one in that frame of mind to go to the rec center. The following are not many fun choices you can attempt to begin with:

Trade out sandwiches for open-confronted sandwiches; removing a portion of the carbs in your sandwich has a gigantic effect on your wholesome equilibrium.

Trade seltzer for soft drinks. You can save more than 20 grams of sugar by making the switch.

Trade Greek yogurt for harsh cream—besides the fact that you save calories, you likewise add solid probiotics to the recipe!

Trade an apple for your bagel—having a morning apple and peanut butter rather than a peanut butter bagel saves calories and carbs and adds supplements to a reasonable eating regimen.

Gradually introduce new behaviors and gradually expand on them.

progress

Building propensities takes time. Show restraint toward yourself and comprehend that the quickest way forward isn't always the most intelligent way forward. The objective of making lifestyle changes isn't to get to the end goal as fast as could be expected. The objective is to assemble propensities that are reasonable in your regular daily existence. Thus, give yourself an opportunity to begin small and expand on progress so the outcome is unshakable.

Track down a way of life, pal.

One of the least demanding ways of making lifestyle changes is to do it with an accomplice! Find a friend who is focused on the interaction and can keep you responsible. This will assist you with considering new propensities to fabricate, keep you inspired, and give you somebody to converse with about the excursion.

Track progress

A simple way to neglect change is by not following advancement. Following advancement is critical to progress, as it shows you how far you've come and where you need to go. Keep tabs on your development so you can learn from difficulties, see normal patterns, and have a pathway to progress.

Transform each conductor in turn.

You don't need to do everything simultaneously! As a matter of fact, it's almost impossible to make lifestyle changes that are built to go the distance, assuming that you are doing them all simultaneously. Making lifestyle changes requires tolerance and commitment. Your cerebrum is mastering another ability and requires time and concentration to construct those neuropathways. Thus, center around building each conduct in turn.

Find out about adjusted nourishment and track down the

equilibrium that works for you.

Each individual's body answers food in an unexpected way, and not all digestion systems work in a very similar way. Cutting calories isn't the best way to get healthy, and as a matter of fact, many eating regimens that cut out whole nutritional categories are unfortunate. Your body needs a good overall arrangement of supplements, including solid fats and carbs. Finding a dietary equilibrium that works for you will assist you in remaining energized and incorporating feasible change into your life.

Track down your why.

Finding your reason is the single most prominent thing you can do to make your way of life change. By finding out what your most profound objective is, you can remain spurred and positive during the interaction. While defining objectives, zeroing in on general wellbeing and lifestyle is useful. Whether your visit is inspired by mathematical pointers, for example, the weight of the executives or the amount you can seat, or by side interests and day-to-day exercises like having the option to run with your companions or play with your grandchildren, finding your most profound reason will assist you with building propensities that last.

Chapter 3:

Beginning with Discontinuous Fast Concerns

Beginning with discontinuous fasting (IF) includes cautious preparation and continuous change. Here are some steps to assist you with starting:

Counsel a Medical Care Proficient:

Prior to beginning any fasting routine, talk with a medical care provider, particularly assuming that you have any hidden ailments or concerns. Choose an IF technique: On the off chance that strategy lines up with your way of life and inclinations, The 16/8 strategy is a well-known beginning stage for some fledglings.

Set your fasting and eating windows:

Decide the hours during which you'll fast and eat. For instance, assuming you pick the 16/8 technique, you could fast from 8:00 p.m. to 12:00 p.m. the following day and eat from 12:00 p.m. to 8:00 p.m. Gradual Change: Begin progressively by moving your feast times closer to your chosen eating window for more than a few days. This assists your body in adjusting to the new schedule.

Pick Supplement Thick Food Sources:

Center around eating whole foods and supplementing thick food sources during your eating window. Incorporate an equilibrium of protein, sound fats, natural products, vegetables, and entire grains. Monitor your body: Focus on how your body answers IF. Certain individuals might encounter introductory yearning or weakness, which can go away as your body adapts. Listen to Your Body: Don't drive yourself too fast in the event that it feels excessively awkward or, on the other hand, assuming that you're encountering unfriendly impacts. Focusing on your wellbeing and prosperity is fundamental.

Remain Predictable:

Consistency is key with IF. Adhere to your chosen plan as intently as could really be expected, yet in addition, permit adaptability for extraordinary events or days when you really want to change your fasting window. Track your advancement: Keep a diary to track your dinners, fasting hours, and how you feel in the meantime. This can assist you in recognizing what works best for you. Be patient: It might take half a month for your body to completely conform to irregular fasting. Show restraint toward yourself and give your body time to adjust.

Screen Your Wellbeing:

Routinely check in with your medical services supplier to guarantee Assuming is appropriate for yourself and not causing any regrettable wellbeing effects. Remember that discontinuous fasting may not be reasonable for everybody, and individual outcomes can shift. It's fundamental to focus on your wellbeing and prosperity and change your fasting routine on a case-by-case basis. On the off chance that you experience any extreme incidental effects, end IF and talk with a medical professional proficient in

Get to know how discontinuous fasting functions.

You don't have to know the full history of IF or the intricate details of every conceivable strategy. We'll get into all the significant stuff later, but for the time being, all you want to know is this:

Discontinuous fasting is the point at which you shift back and forth between times of eating and fasting.

The timetable you pick will determine how long you'll need to prepare and how long you'll need to fit in your feasts and bites.

It's adaptable, and you can change it to suit your life, notwithstanding how occupied and capricious it very well might be!

Pick your fasting plan.

There are different ways of organizing your discontinuous fasting. At Straightforward, we like time-confined eating (TRE) plans, similar to 12/12 and 18/6, best.

The right TRE plan for you will arise as you practice. Our best idea is to begin with 12/12 to consider going all in and perceive how it feels. As you get more experienced, you'll be in a superior position to investigate the other discontinuous fasting choices. If 12/12 feels excessively early, no problem. Essentially, abbreviate your ongoing eating window by 1-2 hours (or whatever amount you're OK with) to expand the time between your last dinner today and your most memorable feast tomorrow.

Counsel your primary care physician.

It's generally smart to check with your primary care physician prior to rolling out a major improvement to how you eat, particularly in the event that you have a background marked by diabetes, coronary illness, or some other ailment. They know you and your wellbeing history, so they'll be very well positioned to guarantee you're protected from the beginning.

An additional note here: Assuming you're presently pregnant or breastfeeding, we don't suggest fasting, as you'll have higher dietary prerequisites that fasting can make hard to meet. You are supporting a somewhat human desire to develop and create, all things considered.

Here are a few signs of discontinuous fasting done well, so you can check in the event that you're on the correct path.

You're quick for 12–18 hours (contingent upon your chosen plan).

This implies you don't eat or drink whatever contains calories for the length of your fasting window. (Look at our aide for the full lowdown on which breaks a quick.)

You consume every one of your calories for the day inside.

6–12 hours (contingent upon your chosen plan).

All that you eat and drink to sustain and empower your body, psyche, and soul squeezes into your eating window.

You adhere to your fasting plan consistently.

Nothing here is permanently established, clearly—in the event that you skirt a day or decide to quick just on specific days of the week, nothing terrible will occur! In any case, to obtain the best outcomes from irregular fasting, consistency is significant, so go day to day if possible.

Your body answers.

At the point when you quick discontinuously, you can anticipate that your body should change here and there, thus:

You might see enhancements in your energy levels over the course of the day.

You might feel more in charge of your hunger.

You might respond better to insulin, particularly in the event that you have a past filled with insulin opposition.

You might feel more engaged to make better food decisions.

Your absorption might improve (more examinations are expected to say without a doubt).

You might shed pounds or creeps from your body.

Once more, you might rest better (more exploration is expected, without a doubt).

Your circulatory strain as well as cholesterol

Obviously, this will be private for you. Sort out what'll let you know that your fasting is working out positively and track those things.

Here and there, it's more straightforward to tell if you're doing it right from what it looks like in the event that you're treating it terribly! Considering that, here are some irregular fasting botches we generally see (no judgment here; these are simple snares to fall into).

You eat when you ought to fast.

That is correct; appetite and desires can steer you off course! This might be an indication that you have picked a fasting plan that is too exhausting or that you're not eating enough during your eating window, so check in with yourself to see what to change.

You quick when you ought to eat

The compulsion to undereat—particularly on the off chance that you're a long-lasting calorie counter—can be a major area of strength. Irregular fasting depends on fasting, but it also depends on you eating what your body needs during your eating window. Support that body!

You get dried out.

Drinking enough is basic when you're discontinuous fasting since you'll probably be eating less. At the point when you eat less, you're likewise getting less water (on the grounds that the food we eat gives us about 33% of the liquid we really want every day). In this way, women should hold back nothing daily, and folks should go for 8–11.

Assuming you notice any side effects of parchedness—like migraines, weariness, or dazedness—that last longer than 24 hours or become unendurable, address your medical care supplier.

You quit when results are slow.

Difficulty, however, substantiates the truth: results are slow. Regardless of whether you're doing everything right, Regardless of whether you're 100 percent committed and every one of your activities is spot-on, Bodies change gradually. Hold tight.

From the beginning, this could appear to be a great deal—so much to ponder and stay away from! We're here to help. Take our basic test and set your fasting plan on the application. From Day 1, we'll stack up articles and experiences to assist you with finishing your diet like a star.

Instructions to Begin Discontinuous Fasting

Certain individuals can flip a switch and hop directly into discontinuous fasting; however, others need to step by step change their eating habits and behaviors. I included myself in that gathering! It took me a half year to take on discontinuous fasting propensities; I was dependent on food, staggering to the storage room for breakfast every morning before I was even conscious.

We're an overloaded country. It's imbued in our minds to have a colossal breakfast and nibble over the course of the day, so it might require investment to adjust to eating less. Perhaps you start irregular fasting on Monday, Wednesday, Friday, or simply toward the end of the week. Whatever seems best for you to start things off

I converse with patients each day who practice responsibility and discipline in their vocations, funds, confidence, and connections; however, food is the one hindrance they battle to control. Discontinuous fasting strips away the intricacies and questions that encompass most other famous weight reduction and health methodologies.

Cut out breakfast

Zane and I could have left your jaw holding tight to the floor during our last discussion when we made sense of the fact that a Grape Nuts business designed the "counsel" that the morning meal is the main dinner of the day.

The best and least demanding method for starting irregular fasting is to remove breakfast from your everyday practice. Your body works its own magic in the first part of the day. Food just hinders it. Cortisol chemicals and adrenals flood in the first part of the day to assist you with awakening, becoming ready, and creating energy.

Why not exploit your body's normal musicality to amplify the advantages of fasting?

Carve out the Best Opportunity to Work Out

Many individuals tragically figure they can't work out while they're fasting; however, the inverse is valid. The morning is the best time for vigorous exercise! You're new and have hormonal improvement on your side.

Evening and night exercises aren't generally really viable; you're exhausted from the day, consumed with anything new that arrived in your lap at work, and are battling the desire to sneak off your shoes and loosen up.

I was faithful to my midday gym routine every day for over 10 years, yet changing to an early morning rec center timetable has been a distinct advantage. In the event that I don't sort it out first thing, I can basically see the sliding scale as I lose my chance over the course of the day for a quality exercise. Life gets going, and the body gets depleted!

Might you at any point drink espresso while

Fasting? (Unwind—you can!)

I understand what you're going to ask with a sprinkle of frenzy in your voice: "Could you at any point actually drink espresso while you're quick?

Indeed! Fortunately for espresso consumers all over the world, our #1 wake-up routine doesn't help our glucose or disturb our quick.

In the event that you can't stomach dark espresso, then indeed, it's alright to add some flavor, but not to an extreme! Remember that your body should consume the fat in the half and half before it can return to consuming your stored fat.

What might be said about espresso consumers who need to veil its harshness with sugar? Zane cautions against every single regular sugar, including natural sweeteners, honey, and agave. The facts confirm that they're "regular" sugars, yet they quickly flood glucose and insulin levels. This thus removes your body from its fasting period through and through.

In the event that you really want a sprinkle of pleasantness in your espresso, stick to a little smidgen of Stevia. Most counterfeit sugars are risky on the grounds that they invigorate desires and stunt your stomach-related framework into getting ready for sugar that isn't coming. This is profoundly troublesome for the fat-consuming cycle that fasting is intended to accomplish.

In general, the subject of espresso relates to your objectives. On the off chance that you're determined to shed 50 pounds, adding cream to your morning blend could slow your progress. However, an improved mug of espresso is obviously superior to a slice of cheesecake! Everything revolves around balance.

Diabetics, fasting is for you as well!

 Zane works consistently with diabetic clients who accept that discontinuous fasting presents an over-the-top gamble.

In any case, as he makes sense of it, "I don't know about a superior method for controlling diabetes or the opposite of those side effects than discovering a good method for presenting fasting."

Type 2 diabetes is an illness of raised glucose, and irregular fasting is an effective method for bringing down and restoring equilibrium glucose levels through better eating techniques.

In my training, I think fasting may very well be the best apparatus my patients need to work on their glycemic control. However long it's cultivated using an essential, specialist-directed plan, diabetics might have the option to utilize fasting to dispense with their dependence on drugs and diminish the impacts of diabetes.

Utilize the Rhythms of Fasting to Timetable Lunch and Supper

You've adequately heard; you're prepared to take a plunge into the brilliant universe of discontinuous fasting. So when, precisely, might you at any point eat?

"The easiest methodology is skipping breakfast and having espresso or tea," Zane frames. Your most memorable feast of the day happens after your fasting period closes, and that implies that all of your eating happens in a compacted window of around six to eight hours.

"That is plus or minus. Make it work with your schedule. Assuming it's six hours, that's amazing. Assuming it must be nine one day, don't pummel yourself," Zane emphasizes.

That is the magnificence of irregular fasting: there's no right. It's one apparatus to work on your wellbeing in a manner that seems OK with your daily practice.

On the off chance that Zane could suggest an ideal irregular fasting plan, this is the very thing he'd propose:

Quit having after supper (8 p.m. at the most recent).

Skip breakfast, partake in your dark espresso or tea, and wait until early afternoon.

Break your fast with a low-carb lunch.

In the event that you really want a bite, make it light.

Partake in a solid supper, then start the quick once more.

 You wouldn't know it from the many "popular" diet and weight reduction books recorded on Amazon; however, further developing your wellbeing doesn't need to be confounded. Pause for a minute to shove aside the messiness in your mind—keto this, sans gluten that. You don't need to bother with a 400-page diet manual to turn your wellbeing around.

Whether you're overweight, diabetic, or excessively occupied for ideal self-care, irregular fasting can bring your body once again into physiological agreement. As a matter of fact, irregular fasting is flooding into ubiquity as additional individuals understand its role as a distinct advantage for weight reduction and health.

Zane Griggs and I had a lot more to investigate after our most memorable discussion about discontinuous fasting, so he has returned to dig further into this rich theme. On the off chance that you're fascinated by irregular fasting but not certain how to incorporate it into your day-to-day daily practice, Zane is here to offer his experiences as an expert wellness mentor, weight reduction mentor, and discontinuous fasting pioneer.

What Characterizes Effective Fasting?

Is fasting simply skipping dinners? Not precisely.

As Zane makes sense of it, "There's more than one method for fasting... By and large, reliance on muscle to fat ratio for fuel begins to be raised after around 12 hours of not taking in that frame of mind of calories."

At its center, discontinuous fasting is basically a 12-hour window between feasts.

So what precisely characterizes effective fasting? Set forth plainly, a fruitful quick method for avoiding your body's way for 12 hours or more As opposed to overburdening your body with food like clockwork, effective fasting offers your body the chance to reset, recalibrate, and consume fat.

The best irregular fasting utilizes a 14- to 18-hour window of no-calorie consumption followed by a 10- to 6-hour window of smart dieting.

Instructions to Begin Discontinuous Fasting

Certain individuals can flip a switch and bounce directly into discontinuous fasting, yet others need to continuously change their eating habits and behaviors. I included myself in that gathering! It took me a half year to embrace discontinuous fasting propensities; I was dependent on food, staggering to the storeroom for breakfast every morning before I was even conscious.

We're an overloaded country. It's imbued in our minds to have a tremendous breakfast and nibble over the course of the day, so it might require investment to adjust to eating less. Perhaps you start discontinuous fasting on Monday, Wednesday, Friday, or simply toward the end of the week. Whatever seems best for you to start things off

I converse with patients each day who practice responsibility and discipline in their vocations, funds, confidence, and connections; however, food is the one deterrent they battle to control. Irregular fasting strips away the intricacies and questions that encompass most other famous weight reduction and wellness methodologies.

Without the veil of disarray, it's not difficult to recognize precisely how to dominate discontinuous fasting and accomplish your objectives.

Cut out breakfast

Zane and I could have left your jaw holding tight to the floor during our last discussion when we made sense of the fact that a grapenut business created the "guidance" that the morning meal is the main feast of the day.

The best and least demanding method for starting discontinuous fasting is to remove breakfast from your everyday practice. Your body works its own sorcery in the first part of the day. Food just hinders it. Cortisol chemicals and adrenals flood in the first part of the day to assist you with awakening, becoming ready, and producing energy.

Why not exploit your body's regular mood to boost the advantages of fasting?

Carve out the Best Opportunity to Work Out

Many individuals tragically figure they can't work out while they're fasting; however, the inverse is valid. The morning is the best time for a fiery workout! You're new and have hormonal enhancement on your side.

Evening and night exercises aren't generally really successful; you're exhausted from the day, consumed with anything new that arrived in your lap at work, and are battling the desire to sneak off your shoes and loosen up.

I was faithful to my midday gym routine every day for over 10 years, yet changing to an early morning exercise center timetable has been a unique advantage. In the event that I don't sort it out first thing, I can essentially see the sliding scale as I lose my chance over the course of the day for a quality exercise. Life gets going, and the body gets depleted!

Could you at any point drink espresso while

Fasting? (Unwind—you can!)

I understand what you're going to ask with a sprinkle of frenzy in your voice: "Could you at any point actually drink espresso while you're quick?

Indeed! Fortunately for espresso consumers all over the world, our number one wake-up routine doesn't help our glucose or disturb our quick.

On the off chance that you can't stomach dark espresso, then indeed, it's alright to add some flavor, but not to an extreme! Remember that your body should consume the fat in the half and half before it can return to consuming your stored fat.

What might be said about espresso consumers who need to cover its sharpness with sugar? Zane cautions against every single regular sugar, including raw sweeteners, honey, and agave. The facts confirm that they're "regular" sugars, yet they quickly flood glucose and insulin levels. This thus removes your body from its fasting period, by and large.

In the event that you want a sprinkle of pleasantness in your espresso, adhere to a little hint of Stevia. Most fake sugars are perilous on the grounds that they animate desires and stunt your stomach-related framework into getting ready for sugar that isn't coming. This is profoundly troublesome for the fat-consuming cycle that fasting is intended to accomplish.

Generally, the subject of espresso relates to your objectives. In the event that you're determined to shed 50 pounds, adding cream to your morning brew could slow your progress. However, an improved mug of espresso is far superior to a slice of cheesecake! Everything revolves around balance.

Diabetics, fasting is for you as well!

Zane works consistently with diabetic clients who accept that discontinuous fasting presents an over-the-top gamble.

However, as he makes sense of it, "I don't know about a superior method for controlling diabetes or conversely, those side effects, other than discovering a smart method for presenting fasting."

Type 2 diabetes is an illness of raised glucose, and discontinuous fasting is a productive method for bringing down and restoring equilibrium glucose levels through better eating systems.

In my training, I think fasting may very well be the best device my patients need to work on their glycemic control. However long it's refined using an essential, specialist-directed plan, diabetics might have the option to utilize fasting to wipe out their dependence on drugs and lessen the impacts of diabetes.

Utilize the Rhythms of Fasting to Timetable Lunch and Supper

You've adequately heard; you're prepared to take a plunge into the superb universe of irregular fasting. So when, precisely, could you at any point eat?

"The easiest methodology is skipping breakfast and having espresso or tea," Zane frames. "In the event that your objective is weight reduction, have a low-carb lunch and supper."

Your most memorable dinner of the day happens after your fasting period closes, and that implies all of your eating happens in a packed window of around six to eight hours.

"That is plus or minus. Make it work with your schedule. On the off chance that it's six hours, fantastic. On the off chance that it must be nine one day, don't pound yourself," Zane underscores.

That is the magnificence of irregular fasting: there's nothing set in stone. It's one apparatus to work on your wellbeing in a manner that seems OK with your daily schedule.

In the event that Zane could suggest an ideal discontinuous fasting plan, this is what he'd propose:

Quit having after supper (8 p.m. at the most recent).

Skip breakfast, partake in your dark espresso or tea, and wait until early afternoon.

Break your fast with a low-carb lunch.

On the off chance that you really want a tidbit, make it light.

Partake in a solid supper, then, at that point, begin the quick once more.

When you feel OK with the rhythm of irregular fasting, you can explore different avenues regarding expanding your quick until 1, 2, or even 3 p.m., all things being equal.

Embrace Dinnertime: People Group

There's a valid reason why a great many people skip breakfast rather than supper. Our nightly feasts are personally friendly and relational. It's been that way since forever! We use supper as a chance to recuperate from our exercises, reconnect with family, and praise the end of one more day. You don't have to deny yourself that rich experience.

All things considered, make a move to practice care as you eat. You'll see the value in each nibble of your food far beyond what you would have expected assuming you'd been eating in your direction as the day progressed. Zane sees this much of the time with his clients: Fasting is best when we keep supper as our center food association.

Eat Toward Your Motivation

We've laid out when to open your mouth during irregular fasting. Yet, when you open your mouth, what precisely would it be advisable for you to eat? There's no right response; everything depends on your objectives.

To shed pounds...

Assuming you're fasting to get more fit, Zane suggests restricting how much starch and sugar you eat. Make this as simple as conceivable by arranging the dinner you'll use every day to break your fast. Wipe out your capacity for indiscreet choices by preparing a delightful, low-carb lunch. Try not to break your quick when the main thing around is Burger Lord.

Supper ought to incorporate lean protein and vegetables; however, adding a solid starch or fat is OK. Keep in mind: You're fulfilling—not rebuffing—yourself with supporting, fulfilling food varieties!

On the off chance that weight reduction isn't your principal objective,

Assuming you're fasting for wellbeing and life span, center around eating genuine food varieties. On the off chance that it wasn't food a long time ago, today's not food! So avoid handled, bundled food varieties and read labels to stay away from the secret snare of added sugars. Everything revolves around an equilibrium of proteins, healthy fats, and veggies. When you enjoy these genuine food varieties, you'll consequently control your intake of those slippery starches.

Attempt 24-Hour Fasting for One Day and Seven Days

Don't confuse yourself over the 24-hour quick. When you're OK with irregular fasting, 24-hour fasting one day a week isn't a major jump.

24-hour fasting is the easiest to begin after supper. Rather than breaking your quick with lunch at 1 p.m., push on for a couple of additional hours to break your quick with supper and festivity.

I can tell you from individual experience from adding this one day a week that the main dinner following a 24-hour quick is so fulfilling. There's nothing else like it—not to mention the fat-consuming and biochemical advantages of giving your body a 24-hour reset.

Deny a Discontinuous Fasting Cheat Day

Zane goes all in on the subject of discontinuous fasting cheat days: "I'm not even certain what the fact is."

A cheat day is comparable to a gorge day for a great many people, yet the impacts of the gorge don't vanish after 24 hours. It can take three or four days to recuperate from the impacts of a cheat day, reign in your desires, recover your energy and concentration, and refocus.

 a lot of hotcakes? Zane inquires. A flood of 1,500 calories of garbage during an irregular fasting cheat day will drive you the other way from your objectives.

Enjoy, don't swindle.

 Revealing is not quite the same as cheating. A little slice of pie or several treats from time to time can assist you with scratching a tingle before you transform into an out-and-out dessert beast.

For the best outcomes, prepare ahead of time. This will hold you back from buckling and giving in each time you have a desire. These extravagances can assist with keeping you propelled and give you state-of mind support.

Be sensible with yourself.

To make discontinuous fasting part of your way of life and arrive at your drawn-out objectives, focus on a timetable and eating design that are feasible for you. If fasting for 18 hours every day and eating low-carb for the remaining six will make you take a lot of cheat days, then perhaps that isn't an ideal timetable for you.

Find what works for your life and focus on it for the long haul.

Irregular fasting can help you in numerous ways, especially with consuming more fat and getting thinner; however, you shouldn't simply go all in. Many individuals battle to begin immediately and improve with slower progress. Investigate these methods for getting into discontinuous fasting at a slower speed for long-haul achievement.

Try not to begin it during another eating regimen.

This is truly significant on the grounds that it can represent the moment of truth in your discontinuous fasting progress. On the off chance that you are doing IF alongside a better approach to eating, such as Keto or a low-calorie diet, you really want to attempt the eating regimen first. Your body needs time to conform to new food sources and dinners, whether you are removing meat from a vegetarian diet or you are diminishing your carbs emphatically. Attempt to adhere to your new eating routine for 14 days, then include irregular fasting. This will make the change go significantly more easily.

Progress Gradually

One more tip that can assist you with progressing into discontinuous fasting is not doing it consistently. This generally applies to fasting conventions like the 16:8 split, where you eat for 8 hours, fast for 16 hours, then recommit the next day. You can in any case acquire benefits from this sort of fasting convention on the off chance that you start with several days per week, have some time off from it, and then, at that point, begin it once more. Consistently, attempt to add on one more day until you can stay with it for the most part. Other fasting conventions, such as 5:2 or Hero, expect you to go an entire 24 hours while fasting, yet you can attempt only 18 or 20 hours, then begin expanding it as you become more comfortable with the fasting window.

Think about your schedule.

This is useful when you are still in the arranging stage and attempting to sort out which irregular fasting convention is ideal for you. You shouldn't pick an event in light of the fact that your companions are making it happen, or you need to attempt the most limit. You truly need to take some real time to contemplate it, checking out your ongoing schedule. Assuming that it is basically impossible that you can have every one of your dinners in only 8 hours in light of a flighty timetable, then the LeanGains 16:8 convention isn't so much for you. Then again, in

the event that you realize you can't complete 24 hours without eating, then it very well may be ideal for you. Consider your inclinations, timetable, and whether it will influence others you live with while deciding which one will be the best fit. This makes that change a lot more straightforward to deal with.

Chapter 4

A Lady's Hormonal Cycle and Irregular Fasting

Irregular fasting is a well-known eating design in which people cycle between times of fasting and eating. While irregular fasting has been shown to have different medical advantages, it is critical to consider what it could mean for a woman's hormonal cycle.

A lady's hormonal cycle is constrained by the period, which comprises a few hormonal vacillations. The two fundamental chemicals included are estrogen and progesterone. Estrogen levels ascend during the follicular stage (before ovulation) and drop during the luteal stage (after ovulation). Progesterone levels increase during the luteal stage to prepare the body for pregnancy.

Discontinuous fasting might possibly influence a lady's hormonal cycle, yet exploration on this subject is restricted. A few examinations recommend that confining calorie consumption or partaking in delayed fasting might upset the feminine cycle or even stop it for a brief time. Nonetheless, a large portion of these examinations have been conducted in creature models or under outrageous fasting conditions.

Irregular fasting is a famous eating design in which people cycle between times of fasting and eating. While discontinuous fasting has been shown to have different medical advantages, it is essential to consider what it could mean for a woman's hormonal cycle.

A lady's hormonal cycle is constrained by the period, which comprises a few hormonal changes. The two fundamental chemicals included are estrogen and progesterone. Estrogen levels ascend during the follicular stage (before ovulation) and drop during the luteal stage (after ovulation). Progesterone levels increase during the luteal stage to prepare the body for pregnancy.

Irregular fasting might possibly influence a woman's hormonal cycle; however, the exploration of this point is restricted. A few studies recommend that limiting calorie consumption or taking part in delayed fasting might disturb the monthly cycle or even stop it briefly. Be that as it may, a large portion of these examinations have been conducted in creature models or under outrageous fasting conditions.

Ladies' hormonal cycles play an urgent role in their general wellbeing and prosperity. These cycles are unpredictably associated with different physiological cycles, including period, richness, and temperament guidelines. Irregular fasting, a dietary methodology acquiring ubiquity, affects ladies' hormonal equilibrium. In this article, we will investigate the connection between discontinuous fasting and women's hormonal cycles. The Rudiments of Ladies' Hormonal Cycles:

Feminine cycle:

The period regularly ranges from 28 days, yet it can change from lady to lady. It comprises four stages: the period, the follicular stage, ovulation, and the luteal phase. Hormones like estrogen and progesterone vary all through this cycle, affecting mindset, energy levels, and ripeness.

Chemicals at Play:

Estrogen:

Predominant in the primary portion of the feminine cycle, it advances egg development and readies the uterine coating for likely pregnancy.

Progesterone:

It becomes the overwhelming focus in the last part, keeping up with the uterine covering and supporting a potential pregnancy. Intermittent Fasting and Ladies' Hormonal Cycles: Irregular fasting includes cycling between times of eating and fasting. While it has shown different medical advantages, its effect on ladies' hormonal cycles is a subject of interest and concern.

Expected Advantages:

Weight The board: Irregular fasting might help weight reduction, which can emphatically influence hormonal balance. Insulin Awareness: It might further develop insulin responsiveness, possibly assisting women with conditions like polycystic ovary disorder. Cellular Wellbeing: Fasting can advance cell autophagy, which could have large wellbeing benefits. Considerations:

Stress Reaction:

Fasting can set off a pressure reaction, prompting expanded cortisol levels. High cortisol levels might upset hormonal balance. Menstrual Inconsistencies: A few ladies might encounter unpredictable periods or missed cycles while rehearsing outrageous fasting.

Individual Fluctuation:

The impacts of discontinuous fasting on women's chemicals can fluctuate generally among individuals. Tips for Ladies Thinking About Irregular Fasting:

Counsel a Medical Services Supplier:

Prior to beginning any fasting routine, talk with a medical care provider, particularly on the off chance that you have basic hormonal issues or are pregnant. Choose a fair methodology: Consider time-limited eating or less outrageous fasting techniques as opposed to delayed diets.

Screen Your Body:

Focus on your body's signs. Assuming that you notice adverse consequences for your period or state of mind, rethink your fasting approach.

End:

Discontinuous fasting can offer likely advantages for ladies, like weight loss and further developed insulin responsiveness. In any case, it's vital to approach it with caution and screen its impacts on your hormonal cycle. Ladies' bodies are exceptional, and what works for one may not work for another. Talking with a medical professional and focusing on your general prosperity ought to be the essential contemplations while exploring different avenues regarding discontinuous fasting.

Investigating the impacts of fasting on chemical

equilibrium and monthly cycle

Fasting, whether explicitly discontinuous or delayed, has been found to affect chemical equilibrium and the period. Here are a few central issues:

Insulin:

Fasting diminishes insulin levels in the body. This can definitely affect chemical equilibrium by lessening insulin obstruction, further developing insulin responsiveness, and possibly assisting with controlling estrogen levels.

Development chemical

Fasting has been shown to promote the creation of development chemicals, which are fundamental for the overwhelming majority of important physical processes. can assist with keeping up with chemical equilibrium by supporting the development of different chemicals, for example, insulin-like development factor and thyroid chemicals.

Leptin

Leptin is a chemical created by fat cells that manages hunger and digestion. Discontinuous fasting has been associated with improved leptin awareness, which can emphatically impact hormonal guidelines and monthly cycle routineness.

Cortisol

Fasting can at first cause an expansion in cortisol levels, particularly when joined by calorie restriction. Fasting can affect chemical equilibrium and the feminine cycle, yet it is important to take note that singular reactions can differ. A few potential impacts include: Changes in Insulin Levels: Fasting might prompt lower insulin levels, which can influence different chemicals like leptin and adiponectin. This can affect feminine regularity. Stress Chemicals: Broadened fasting or inordinate calorie limitation can set off the arrival of stress chemicals like cortisol, possibly disturbing the feminine cycle. Amenorrhea: Serious fasting or outrageous caloric limitation can prompt amenorrhea, the shortfall of feminine periods. This is often found in people with eating disorders. Hormone irregular characteristics: Fasting could influence chemicals like luteinizing chemicals and follicle-animating chemicals, which are urgent for ovulation and menstruation. Body Fat Rate: Fasting can diminish muscle versus fat, which might affect estrogen levels since estrogen is created in fat

tissue. This can influence the feminine cycle.
Adaptation: A few ladies might adjust to
discontinuous fasting without huge hormonal
interruptions. Momentary fasting, also known as
discontinuous fasting, may not influence the
feminine cycle for everyone. It's vital to
approach fasting with alertness, particularly for
ladies of conceptual age. Talk with a medical
care supplier or an enrolled dietitian prior to
beginning any fasting routine, as they can give
direction custom-made to your particular
requirements and screen any possible impacts on
your chemical equilibrium and feminine cycle.
Checking your body's reaction and maintaining a
fair, supplement-rich eating regimen is essential
for general wellbeing, including feminine
wellbeing.

Changing your fasting routine to help hormonal wellbeing

If you are fasting and need to help your
hormonal wellbeing, moving toward fasting in a

fair and economical way is significant. Here are a few hints:

Timing: Consider changing your fasting window

to line up

with your normal circadian cadence.

This implies fasting during hours when your body is normally prepared for fasting, for example, in the short term. This can assist with directing your body's inward clock and restoring hormonal equilibrium.

Calorie consumption:

Guarantee that you are consuming an adequate number of calories during your non-fasting periods. Serious calorie limitation can disturb chemicals and adversely influence feminine cycle consistency. Pay attention to your body's craving signs and ensure you are eating an adequate number of sustaining food varieties.

Macronutrients:

Center around including an assortment of macronutrients in your eating regimen during non-fasting periods. This implies consuming an equilibrium of carbs, proteins, and solid fats, as they all assume significant roles in chemical creation and guidance.

In the event that you're thinking about changing your fasting routine to help with hormonal wellbeing, here are a few rules to consider: Consult a medical service proficient: Prior to rolling out any improvements to your fasting schedule, talk with a medical care supplier or an enlisted dietitian who has some expertise in ladies' wellbeing. They can give customized direction in view of your particular necessities and wellbeing status. Choose a maintainable fasting example: Rather than outrageous fasting, decide on additional moderate methodologies like discontinuous fasting. This can include everyday time-confined eating windows (e.g., the 16/8 strategy) or incidental fasting days as opposed to delayed fasting.

Keep away from inordinate caloric limitations:

Guarantee that you're actually consuming an adequate number of calories to meet your energy needs and maintain a healthy body weight. Outrageous calorie limitations can upset chemical equilibrium.

Focus on Supplement Thick Food Varieties:

Center around a decent eating routine rich in entire food sources, including natural products, vegetables, lean proteins, and sound fats. Sufficient admission of fundamental supplements upholds hormonal wellbeing.

Screen Protein Admission:

Satisfactory protein is fundamental for chemical union and general wellbeing. Ensure you're getting sufficient, excellent protein sources in your eating regimen.

Remain Hydrated:

Appropriate hydration is essential for hormonal equilibrium and general prosperity. Hydrate over the course of the day. Manage stress: Constant pressure can upset chemicals. Consolidate pressure-reducing strategies like care, yoga, or reflection into your daily schedule.

Focus on Macronutrients:

The equilibrium of starches, fats, and proteins in your eating regimen can affect chemicals. Explore different avenues regarding different macronutrient proportions to see what works best for you.

Pay attention to your body:

Focus on how your body responds to fasting. On the off chance that you notice adverse consequences for your monthly cycle, energy levels, or temperament, consider changing your fasting design or consulting a medical services professional.Supplement Carefully: A few ladies might benefit from explicit enhancements to help hormonal wellbeing, like omega-3 unsaturated fats or certain nutrients and minerals. Examine supplementation with a medical care provider. Remember that singular reactions to fasting can change, and what works for one individual may not work for another. Focusing on your general wellbeing and prosperity over severe adherence to a fasting regimen is fundamental. Normal registrations with a medical services supplier can assist you in settling on informed conclusions about your fasting routine and its effect on hormonal wellbeing.

Chapter 5

The science behind discontinuous fasting

Discontinuous fasting (IF) is an eating design that shifts back and forth between times of fasting and eating. The science behind discontinuous fasting is perplexing, yet here are some vital points: Insulin Guideline: Fasting periods can bring down insulin levels, making muscle and fat more open for energy. This might support weight reduction.

Autophagy:

During fasting, cells start a cycle called autophagy, where they eliminate damaged parts and reuse them. This is known to have different medical advantages.

Chemical Guideline:

IF can influence the arrival of chemicals like ghrelin (a hunger chemical) and leptin (a satiety chemical), possibly diminishing general calorie intake. Cellular Fix: Fasting triggers cell fix processes, which can upgrade life span and decrease the risk of ongoing sickness.

Metabolic Advantages:

That's what a few investigations recommend: IF can further develop insulin responsiveness, lessen irritation, and advance better glucose control.

Weight of the board:

On the off chance that it might assist with weight reduction by creating a calorie deficit and expanding fat oxidation. Brain Wellbeing: There's proof that IF could uphold cerebrum wellbeing, including mental capability and a diminished risk of neurodegenerative illnesses.

Heart Wellbeing:

IF may work on cardiovascular wellbeing by diminishing risk factors like circulatory strain, cholesterol levels, and triglycerides. It's critical to take note of the fact that while there's promising research on irregular fasting, individual reactions can change. Prior to beginning an IF routine, talk with a medical professional, particularly on the off chance that you have basic ailments. It's fundamental to guarantee that Assuming is protected and appropriate for your particular conditions.

Science

You've presumably heard the publicity: discontinuous fasting has been hailed as the key to weight reduction.

In any case, what's the truth?

While there is believable logical proof for irregular fasting's

advantages, it's neither a speedy nor a surefire fix, as indicated by driving scientist Satchin Panda.

Panda, a teacher of circadian science at the Salk Foundation for Organic Examinations in La Jolla, California, has spent his vocation concentrating on the complex biochemical cycles of the human body. His examination—in mice and individuals—suggests that irregular fasting could help human wellbeing in a wide range of ways, including getting in shape.

Before we plunge into the science, how about we put one thing front and center: There's no method for doing discontinuous fasting. In the event that you Google it, you'll track down a menu of choices, each with their own defenders. There's the 5:2 eating routine, which includes eating not many calories (approximately 500–600) for two days of the week, followed by five days of ordinary eating. On the other hand, there's other-day fasting, which implies eating regularly one day and then eating either nothing or only 500 calories the following.

All discontinuous fasting strategies are basically founded on

a similar thought: When you decrease your caloric intake, your body will use its stored fat for energy.

However, what makes irregular fasting not quite the same as basically cutting calories is the likelihood that it's simpler for individuals to confine calories to restricted time frames instead of for the long stretches of time requested by traditional weight control plans. Furthermore, the particular sort of irregular fasting that Panda has considered may have additional impacts.

Panda has zeroed in on a discontinuous fasting technique known as time-confined eating.

In this organization, an individual consumes every one of their calories for the day within an 8-to-12-hour window. Suppose you typically start your day with a first mug of espresso at 7 a.m. and, at last, wind down with popcorn and a beverage around 11 p.m. With time-limited eating, you could change to having breakfast at 8 a.m., including espresso, and completing your supper by 6 p.m. Like that, you're eating every one of your dinners within a 10-hour window—and you're doubtlessly renouncing calories from pastries, evening tidbits, and liquor.

Time-confined eating is, by all accounts, accomplishing more for the body than basically lessening calorie intake. This was first proposed in a recent report that Panda and partners did with mice. They took two hereditarily indistinguishable arrangements of mice and gave them a similar eating regimen—a lab-mice form of the standard American eating regimen that is high in fat and straightforward sugar and low in protein.

While the two gatherings were given precisely the same measure of food, one gathering received nourishment for 24 hours and the other for just 8 hours. Mice are nighttime creatures, ordinarily dozing during the day and eating around evening time. In any case, when one gathering was given nonstop access to food, those mice begged

Following 18 weeks, the mice could eat at an extremely

inconvenient times gave indications of insulin obstruction and, furthermore, had liver harm.

Yet the mice who ate in an 8-hour window didn't have these circumstances. They likewise weighed 28%, not exactly the mice with 24-hour access to food, despite the fact that the two groups of mice ate a similar number of calories daily. "It was somewhat momentous," Panda says. Up to that point, he says that he and different scientists had thought that the complete number of calories, as opposed to when they were eaten, resolved weight gain.

His group rehashed the investigation with three extra arrangements of mice and came up with similar outcomes. The results likewise held consistent for various sorts of food and for gobbling windows of as long as 15 hours—albeit, curiously, the more limited the window, the less weight the mice acquired. At the point when the time-confined mice were switched over to unhindered eating for two days every week, or what Panda calls "having the end of the week off", they actually put on less weight than the mice permitted to eat 24 hours per day.

Then, Panda's group additionally attempted it another way: they took mice that had put on weight on account of unlimited care and changed them to time-confined eating. Notwithstanding eating similar amounts of calories, these mice shed pounds and kept up with it for a very long time for the rest of the review. They additionally diminished their insulin obstruction, which is believed to be connected to corpulence, despite the fact that researchers actually don't figure out the affiliation. Obviously, the human body is more complicated than that of a mouse, Panda says, yet these tests were the principal sign of how significant timing could be with regards to how our bodies use food.

Lately, researchers have been finding that so many of the

The human body's cycles are attached to our circadian rhythms. For instance, the greater part of us know that getting daylight promptly toward the beginning of the day is helpful to our temperament and rest and that being presented to light at 9 p.m. through our PDAs or workstations can disturb our night's rest. Rather than being utilized as fuel, it gets put away as fat, which appears to be legit once you analyze the nuts and bolts of how human digestion functions.

Time-limited eating gives our body additional opportunities to burn fat. At the point when we eat, our body involves sugars for energy, and in the event that we don't require them immediately, they get put away in the liver as glycogen or changed over into fat. After we've gotten done eating for the afternoon, our body keeps running on glucose from the sugars that we've recently eaten for a couple of hours prior to taking advantage of stored starches, or glycogen, in the liver. That glycogen goes on for a few hours prior to running out approximately eight hours after we've quit eating, which is the point at which our body starts to take advantage of its stored fat.

At the point when we abbreviate our eating window and

As we expand our fasting window, we spend longer in this fat-consuming method of digestion.

Be that as it may, the second we ingest food once more—regardless of whether it's only espresso with a touch of sugar and milk—we switch once more into the other mode and begin consuming starches and putting away glycogen and fat. So assuming that you complete the process of eating

at 10 p.m. with your nightly nibble, your body
will run out of glycogen and begin consuming
fat at around 6 a.m.Assuming you generally have
breakfast at 6 a.m., if you change that to 9 a.m.,
you've given your body an additional three hours
to use fat as fuel.

Panda followed up on his time-limited eating tests with people.

and found it showed a guarantee there as well.

In 2015, he and his partners took a stab at
putting Little Gathering on a period-limited
eating plan for quite some time. Intriguingly, the
scientists offered these individuals no eating
regimen directions or guidance by any means.
All things being equal, the subjects were told to
pick a 10- to 12-hour window in which to do all
their eating. At the point when they ate, they
took photos of their food and messaged them to
the specialists. Following four months, the
subjects showed a modest quantity of weight

reduction—a normal of a little more than 8 pounds each. Be that as it may, they detailed encountering better rest, more energy in the mornings, and less yearning at sleep time, recommending time-limited eating, which "really has a foundational influence all around the body," as per Panda. While it was excessively little to have the option to reach conclusive inferences, the scientists found it empowering that this straightforward intercession appeared to be simple for subjects to execute and support

Final summary

Irregular fasting is a dietary methodology where people switch back and forth between times of fasting and eating. It has acquired prevalence because of its potential medical advantages and adequacy for weight reduction. This article gives a rundown of "how to flourish" while rehearsing irregular fasting, suggesting that the emphasis will be on boosting the advantages and guaranteeing a good outcome with this eating design.

Flourishing with irregular fasting (IF) as a lady includes counseling a medical care professional for security, picking a reasonable IF strategy, bit by bit changing, remaining hydrated, keeping up with adjusted sustenance, focusing on protein, being aware of chemicals, taking supplements into account, observing advancement, overseeing rest and stress, and embracing consistency and persistence in your methodology. Customization and expert direction are fundamental to the outcome of IF.